An Educational Guide to Healthy Hair
How to Obtain and Maintain a Healthy Head of Hair

By Melva Williams

An Educational Guide to Healthy Hair:
How to Obtain and Maintain a Healthy Head of Hair
First Edition, April 2015

Mended Tresses
Irving, Texas

Author: Melva Williams

Specials thanks to the team at Curiouser Editing:
Shayla Eaton, editor
Rodrigo Sabillon, illustrator
Jessica Allée, formatter
www.curiousediting.com

Endorsements

As editor in chief of *Enticing Resultz Magazine,* I have had my fair share of reading material. I have interviewed some prominent people in the hair and beauty industry. I must say that when approached by a publicist hailing from the opposite side of the country to get me an interview with a hairstylist in Texas by the name of Melva Williams, I thought, *Sure, we would exchange a few words of hairstyling from a great celebrity hairstylist.* But during our rapport, I understood the business acumen that this woman possessed.

She was a mogul in the making. I can actually say that I have witnessed her growth in a short while, even though she has been building her dreams for countless years. It's women like Melva Williams—hairstylist, salon owner, author—who continue to inspire me. I also have a long track record of business and entrepreneurial skills to say the least. As a licensed hairstylist and salon owner, nurse and community health educator, I could understand the need for a book that spoke volumes but in a manner that everyone could understand. I also had a chance to sample some of Melva's product line personally delivered to my salon in New York. I was very impressed, and so were my clients. And of course, I followed up with a product review in the publication as well.

I must admit that Melva is one of the most humble people that I know. She has the knowledge and experience that we as hairstylists need. She isn't afraid to say what you need to hear.

Health is wealth. She knows this and teaches this quite fervently to her clients as well as other stylists. Her teachings are what appealed to me, because I also teach the same to my clients.

If you are a hairstylist and wonder, "How do I communicate the needs of my clients versus their wants? How do I express to them that healing starts on the inside of them, followed by regularly scheduled appointments? How do I incorporate healthy products into my regime?" then this book is for you.

After reading, you will feel more confident that you will have the knowledge to go forth and become a successful hairstylist and step your game up to the pros. This will help you not only to be a good stylist but a great one!

Shanell Monique

Enticing Resultz Magazine, Editor in Chief

www.shanellmonique.com

www.enticingresultz.com

~*~

As an African-American woman, I have struggled over the years with maintaining a healthy head of hair. I have spent many years reading magazines and using products that were just not the right fit for me. I have gone in between natural and relaxed hair, not able to figure out the reason why I could not maintain beautiful hair.

As the CEO of Power Forward Woman, I had to begin to really take my looks seriously because of my direct relationship with women and the public. One day, I ran across a woman with a great spirit by the name of Melva Williams. I had no idea that she was a hairstylist during our first meeting, but as our relationship grew, I could see the passion that she had for hair.

The amazing thing about Melva Williams is that she is more than just hair but a prominent business woman who not only has the passion to spread her movement about healthy hair but also a passion to empower, encourage, and educate women about it. She is more than just a stylist; she is a woman on a mission!

Melva Williams is a phenomenal woman and touches the hearts of everyone that she comes into contact with. Her ability to transform her clients' hair and also educate them on how to maintain healthy hair is nothing short of amazing. I believe that her teachings will allow women across America to be able to connect the dots and truly understand that having healthy hair is more than just a routine—it's truly knowing your health.

After reading this book, I'm sure that Melva Williams, the educator, the stylist, and the Power Forward Woman, will have helped millions of women change their thoughts about hair.

Star Williams, CEO

Power Forward Woman

"Because of a strong you, we become a stronger US, United Sisters."

star@powerforwardwoman.com

www.facebook.com/Powerforwardwoman

www.twitter.com/PowerForwardWom

www.powerforwardwoman.com

~*~

As an African-American woman, a breast cancer survivor, and a mentor for a social network survivors' group, I see firsthand the devastating effects of cancer treatments on our hair. After all, we were raised to regard our hair as our crown of glory.

From a very young age, many African-American ladies start manipulating and stressing the hair with added hair, wigs, and perms for vanity purposes mostly, as with most women. We often see in fashion magazines, on television, and in fashion images everywhere all the hype about creative hairstyling without any knowledge of hair health.

Throughout our lifetime, curveballs are thrown at us such as stress, career changes, and compromised health, to name a few, which all have an effect on our hair. I was never educated on how my hair health is impacted by these life changes. I also was not aware that I could do things to reverse some of the harmful damage it has caused.

From the very first visit to Melva Williams, over ten years ago, she started enlightening me about proper hair care. When I was diagnosed with breast cancer, my hair salon visits, as you can imagine, were put on hold. After harsh breast cancer treatments, I came back to Melva and it was a true blessing to know that she was armed and ready to educate me and my fellow survivors on how we can take control over our hair health.

When she shared with the ladies in my social network group how everything we ingest from food and medicine to our daily activity levels all play a role in how our hair grows, the ladies felt empowered and their hope was restored.

I feel that both men and women, of any race or culture, will find this information in this *Educational Guide to Healthy Hair* to be helpful and relevant in their quest for healthy hair. This comprehensive book is based on her critical analysis and research. It addresses the anecdotes and consequences that offer practical strategies for promoting hair wellness and recovery.

I extend my appreciation and gratitude to Melva Williams for offering a solution that is measurable and easy to understand.

Leslie Y. Williams, CEO

Survivors On Purpose, Inc.

www.survivorsonpurpose.com

lwilliams@survivorsonpurpose.com

www.facebook.com/survivorsonpurpose

Acknowledgments

I would like to dedicate this book to Ryan Williams, my loving husband, soul mate, business partner, and best friend. You have stood by my side, pushed, pulled, invested, persuaded, advised, and consoled me all when I have desperately needed it. I could not have done any of this without you. We have so much more ground to cover, and the journey has just begun. There is a bigger picture being painted in our lives. I owe you and God so much.

To my devoted clients, followers, products users, team, and those in the past and present: thank you for always supporting me, inspiring me, praying for me, challenging me, and encouraging me. I hope you know the value that you will always hold in my life.

To Sonya Eiland and Theresa Martin: thank you for giving so unselfishly of yourselves. You helped to write the blueprint in the beginning of my journey freely from your heart. I will forever be grateful to you. I thank God for crossing our paths.

Table of Contents

Chapter 6: Unmasking a Woman's Hidden Beauty

Introduction

After being in the beauty industry for twenty-four years, I felt compelled to give my clients more than a beautiful head of hair. I have come in to contact with many women who have issues from medical problems, improper dieting, lack of exercise, medication, stress, hormones, metabolism, and dehydration. Over ten years ago, I began to research how I could help these women with their hair. I realized that every woman is not going to come into the salon with a beautiful, healthy head of hair.

As my life seemed to unravel and research progressed, it seems as though I had needed this information for myself and that made my research even more intense. I never would've imagined that all these internal things affecting our everyday lives also affect our hair loss or growth.

As I began to share with my clients and counsel them about their hair, they had never heard these things before. They stated that a stylist had never asked them these things. Some even asked me, "What does that have to do with my hair?" They followed the instructions and saw major results in their hair.

Women who had bald spots for years saw their hair grow back. Women who said their hair would never grow now have hair. Women who had issues growing their hair and stated it would grow to a certain length and break off now have the longest hair they've ever had before.

I knew that I had to share this information with the world because it was too important to keep it to myself.

A woman is only as beautiful as she feels from the inside out, but sometimes she recognizes an attribute from the outside. Her hair is one of those attributes. A woman's hair is an extension of the very essence of sensuality. It makes her feel a certain way. When her hair is sick, she is too. When she's not feeling quite herself, she gets her hair done and feels like a new person.

This book is for women of all ages, cultures, races, and hair textures. It's for women all over the world with medical issues; for women on medication; for women who are stressed or have hormone and metabolism problems—it's for women who want healthy hair. For every woman who wants to understand how diet and exercise affects her hair. This book is to help women connect the dots to see how their medical issues and hair issues relate to each other.

For the mother who wants to learn how to grow her daughter's hair. For the stylist who wants to learn about healthy hair—she doesn't have to reinvent the wheel. For the student before she ever finishes school and touches her first head of hair. This is for all women; they now know what it takes to have a healthy head of hair.

Everything starts from the inside out—especially having a healthy head of hair.

Chapter 1: A Successful Formula for Healthy Hair

Getting to Know Your Stylist

As you have heard, a hair-care professional is a counselor, priest, and friend. We wear many hats. But at the end of the day, the one that proves most important is stylist.

If you have a stylist, she (or he) needs to know your styling likes or dislikes, your profession, your lifestyle, and your environment influences that may affect your hair. Informed with this information, your stylist can provide easier and faster service. You do not have to go over your list of likes or dislikes at each visit. Even if you ask for a different style, a stylist will know how to change it to your liking.

Knowing your clients' professions is important. If you are a business professional and you ask for a color change of red, the stylist would know not to give you a bright-red color. If someone is very modest in her appearance, the stylist will not give her a style that would draw attention to her. As you know, these changes for these two very different types of women would not fit their profession or appeal to them emotionally. (This comes from not knowing your client.)

Here are questions that are important in looking for a stylist. In your search, you should be interviewing them as well to see if they are a fit for you.

Five Important Questions to Ask Your Stylist:
1. What type of products do you use?
2. What services do you specialize in?
3. What are your hours of operation?
4. What are your prices?
5. What is your cancellation policy?

It's important to know the answers to these questions, so take the time to talk to your stylist. Things you may not consider to be important may prove to be valuable later on.

Even if you are not a regular at the salon, the stylist should be listening fully to what you want, to your likes and dislikes, and asking questions before beginning your service to ensure a proper outcome.

You Want Me to Do What to Your Hair?

When a client steps into the salon, most of the time she has somewhat of a vision; but there are a few who have a dream. The ones who have the vision have been thinking of this style for a while. They have been seeing it in their head, looking at the picture over and over again. It does not matter if they have enough hair for it; if their hair is healthy enough for it, they just want the stylist to create it. After all, the stylist is the magician. (Like it or not, that's what I am!)

There is a responsibility attached with this title that I supposedly hold a special wand to perform magic tricks with.

When a client with damaged, dry hair asks for color in my salon, there is no way this is going to happen. If she is a referral who wants color, the referring client will tell her, "She's not going to give you color. You don't drink water."

This is a need versus want. I will consult with the client and let her know she needs to properly hydrate herself and that if I gave her color, she would not be happy with it. Giving a permanent color at this time would further dry out her hair and could cause it to break due to lack of moisture and elasticity.

I'm honest with the client, telling her all the reasons why I will not give her the service she wants; then I explain what she needs to do in order to get the service later on down the line. The client is happy with this honest report instead of my damaging her hair; I have gained the client's trust and her business for a long time. I have also fulfilled my responsibility to give the client what she needs versus what she wants.

It is my responsibility to say, "No, that is not a good idea." Some clients have even walked out the door and walked back in because they realized that my hair guidelines are essential to hair maintenance, development, and growth.

Why It's a Team Effort

Two heads are always better than one, unless they are on the same person. But when it comes to the stylist and client, this duo makes a great team.

The stylist can only do her part at the salon, and the client can only do her part at home; but they are both important. If the stylist is using great products, the right tools, asking all the right questions, educating herself, then she is doing her part. On the other hand, if the client is failing to wrap her hair at night, drink water, or take vitamins and the stylist and client are not communicating, this makes it even worse.

If a client has any medical issues, takes medications, or has surgeries coming up, your stylist should know because all of these things affect hair. This is in accordance to quite a few medical reviews. One review found by Lindsey Marcellin, MD, MPH (Masters in Public Health), in a 2011 book, *When Hair Loss Is Not Genic,* by Krisha McCroy.

Most times when clients are in the chair at the salon, things regarding their health may need to be discussed but are often not. Both stylist and client have an important role to play in ensuring hair health consistency is the key.

Chapter 2: Medical Influences

So many women today have medical issues and are losing their hair, but they have not connected the dots that the two are related. Here in this chapter, I want to help shed some light on some areas that many of you may not be aware of. By being aware of this, the client can now decide if she wants or needs to go to natural hair and the stylist will know to use a lighter chemical (teamwork).

Effects of Medication and Medical Issues

Certain drugs interfere with the hairs' normal growth cycle, allowing the follicles to go into a resting phase for a longer period. It prevents the matrix cells from making new hairs, more so in cancer patients.

According to WebMD 2005–2013, here is a list of medications that cause hair loss:
- Acne medications containing vitamin A (retinoid)
- Antibiotics and antifungal drugs
- Anticlotting drugs
- Antidepressants
- Birth control pills
- Cholesterol-lowering drugs
- Drugs that suppress the immune system
- Drugs that treat breast cancer
- Epilepsy drugs (anticonvulsants)
- High blood pressure medications (anti-hypertensive), such as beta-blockers, ACE inhibitors, and diuretics
- Hormone replacement therapy
- Mood stabilizers
- Parkinson's disease drugs

- Steroid
- Thyroid medication

Always check medications for side effects for yourself and by consulting your doctor. The best way to determine if it is truly the medication is to assess where you were before the medication (must be an honest account). After about three to four months, if your hair is still breaking, dry and brittle, or having follicle damage and if there is no change, ask your doctor if there is an alternative medication. But be careful, side effects may be no different or worse.

Tell your stylist if you are having surgery and going under anesthesia. Remember that anything entering your bloodstream will affect your hair. So after surgery, you will notice some shedding.

Stress Factors

Back in the day, I had always heard that stress was the number one cause of hair loss. We have so much on our plates today that I can see why the hair market is on the rise as a number one selling market. This hair loss factor is not permanent; however, it is very important.

There are three different types of stress factors according to Dr. Daniel K. Hall-Flavin, MD:

- *Alopecia areata.* A variety of factors are thought to cause alopecia areata, possibly including severe stress. With alopecia areata, white blood cells attack the hair follicle, stopping hair growth and making hair fall out.

- *Telogen effluvium.* In this condition, emotional or physical stress pushes large numbers of growing hairs into a resting phase. Within a few months, the affected hairs may fall out suddenly when simply combing or washing your hair.

- *Trichotillomania.* Trichotillomania (trik-oh-til-oh-MAY-nee-uh) is an irresistible urge to pull out hair from your scalp, eyebrows, or other areas of your body. Hairpulling can be a way of dealing with negative or uncomfortable feelings, such as stress, anxiety, tension, loneliness, fatigue, or frustration.

If this is a really important issue that you feel you need to seek medical help for, then please do so; but there are others way in dealing with stress that will also help your hair.

Regular exercise at least three to four times a week can promote hair growth. According to Revivogen.com, when you are stressed, it's possible for your hair to thin or fall out. Stress tends to produce a hormone called *cortisone* that causes the growth of the hair follicles. This type of stress can result in the hair beginning to thin over time. Cardiovascular exercise can reduce the amount of cortisone present in the body. These lower levels of the cortisone hormone decrease over time and will help hair grow faster and fuller.

With exercise, you will decrease your stress. This will increase the serotonin levels in your brain, which will lower cortisone in the body. Over time, you will begin to view life in a different way, feeling happier and creating balance. The whole body is affected when you are under an extreme amount of stress. Exercise can help reduce stress and promote hair growth at the same time.

Hormones

Hormonal changes in the body affect hair loss or growth. These changes determine whether growth stops, how much grows, and if new hair grows. This process can also cause abnormal growth as well. This explains that hair has grown awry.

The hormones with the most direct effect on hair growth are androgens, the male sex hormones that include testosterone. These androgens are found in both men and women; one gender just produces more than the other because of the testosterone factor. Due to these androgens, they are the contributing factor in male and female pattern baldness. This factor prevents hair follicles from transitioning out of its normal resting phase. An overproduction of androgens causes women to have excessive facial and body hair. The University of Maryland Medical Center notes the reason for this is unclear.

But there are natural ways to help balance your hormones and help your hair at the same time.

1. *Changing your diet will help your hormones levels.*

- Zinc has been known to lower hormone levels and help in the production of testosterone. Foods found to be high in zinc include dark chocolate, peanuts, and many meats, including beef, veal, lamb, crab, and oysters.
- You can also try eating foods high in omega-3 fatty acids. These fatty acids create healthy membranes, which allow hormones to reach their desired destination within our bodies. Some foods that include omega-3 are walnuts, eggs, and many types of fish, including sardines, trout, salmon, tuna, and oysters.
- Include more fiber in your diet. High-fiber foods include whole grains, raw fruit, and raw vegetables. Fiber helps to regulate your system by releasing old estrogen. This release will help to create balance in your digestive system and help to regulate hormones.
- Avoid excessive use caffeine and alcohol. This has been known to contribute to premenstrual hormonal imbalance.

2. Exercise more often.

- Cardiovascular exercise has been known to release serotonins. These chemicals decrease mood swings and also help with the female reproductive hormones.

3. Reduce stress.

- A loss of estrogen is linked to mood disorders in women. This happens with excess stress because of lowered serotonin levels. Remember: exercise helps to release these serotonins.

Chapter 3: How to Grow Out Hair Properly

I've covered what I believe to be a successful formula for healthy hair, medical influences, and matters that affect the hair growth. Now I would like to give you the technique that I have watched over the years work successfully in properly growing out hair.

Trimming, Treatments, and Time

This technique may not seem like a technique at all, but if you do any kind of research, you will notice these are proven facts. You can do some methods (not all of them) and get some results. But if you do them all in combination, like anything else, you will receive maximum results.

Trimming

Hair should be trimmed at least six to eight weeks to ensure proper growth. Hair grows at different speeds from person to person. Some people have hair that grows quickly, while others have hair that grows slower. Some people have sections of hair that grow quicker than others, causing a carefully maintained haircut to become choppy at the ends. Frequent trims help keep your hair at a desired length and prevent your layers from looking untamed.

Trimming your hair makes a difference in keeping your haircut looking well maintained. It keeps your hair fresh and healthy. Getting rid of split ends allows hair to grow faster. Not trimming the unhealthy ends and leaving them to continue to split further actually does more damage. Your ends continue to split, and you end up needing more trimmed. Just make sure to stick to one hairstylist who knows what you like to prevent going for a trim and walking out with four inches chopped off your locks.

Treatments focus on more than just one main area of the hair and go a bit deeper into the hair shaft than a normal conditioner. Regular conditioner when you have a major hair issue is like putting a Band-Aid on an open wound. Also, if the issue is internal, it will only get worse. (This can be under one of the medical influences.) That's why the hair will continue to shed until the hair is treated properly. Most treatments you buy in a beauty supply store are not strong enough. You have to contact a salon professional about stopping breakage if the breakage is severe.

There are different types of treatments depending on what the hair needs.

For hair that is weak—shedding and breaking—it will most likely need protein and amino acids for strength.

Hair that is dry, brittle, has no luster, and has lost moisture either needs hot oil treatment, vitamin E, fortifier, keratin, protein with vitamin B5, or antioxidants.

Time

Hair has three growth cycles. Getting a better understanding of this will help you with knowing how to properly grow out your hair.

1. *Anagen*

   This is where the hair growth cycle begins. Normally, up to 90 percent of the hair follicles are in the anagen phase. During this phase, cells in the root of the hair divide, adding to the hair shaft, and grow about one centimeter every twenty-eight days. The cycle's length varies for different parts of the body. Scalp hair stays in this active phase for two to six years. The growth cycle is controlled by a chemical signal like epidermal growth factor, which is a factor that stimulates cell growth.

2. *Catagen*

   The catagen is the involution or the regressing phase. Normally, 1 to 2 percent of the hair follicles are in the catagen phase. This is a short transitional period where the hair is no longer growing. This happens at the end of the anagen phase and signals the end of the active growth of a hair. This phase lasts for two or three weeks, and during this, a club hair is formed. The club hair allows the hair follicle to be cut off from its blood supply and the cells that produce new hair when a club hair occurs when the section of the follicle attaches to the hair shaft.

3. *Telogen*

The final stage of the hair growth and shedding cycle is the telogen or resting phase. During this two- to four-month phase, the hair begins to shed at normal levels and the anagen phase begins again producing new hair. This is the final and resting stage of the hair growth cycle. This cycle could last up to two to four months and at least fifty to one hundred club hairs are shed daily. After this cycle, the anagen phase begins producing new hair.

Again, it is important for your stylist to know these stages and to know his or her client and recognizing which stage they may be in. It may not be wise to get a haircut while the hair is in its resting phase, because it may seem like it takes forever for it to grow back.

Diet and Exercise

So many times we have heard, "You are what you eat," but who really cares about this when it comes to their hair? After all, what do the two have to do with each other?

There are foods that our bodies need plenty of and that help our hair. But if we are lacking certain foods, it can hurt us as well. As the doctors have always said, "Diet and exercise go hand-in-hand." When you exercise, you stimulate the blood flow in your scalp. These two in combination are a great addition to growing out your hair.

Diet

Hair is made of protein. All basic nutrients contribute to keeping us whole and healthy. All the basic nutrients provide wholeness that keeps us healthy. Mainly, protein supplies us with building blocks that repair and replace skin, muscles, bone growth, and hair. When you say *protein*, I think most people think meats: steak, fish, chicken. But there are many other sources of dietary protein such as eggs, dairy products, soy foods, whole grains, and vegetables. Be careful, though! In smaller amounts, too much of a good thing can show up as bulk.

There are some people who lack protein in their diets, and it shows up in their hair, such as those with anorexia nervosa or those who follow extreme weight loss diets. These diets will slow the rate of new hair growth, pushing the hair into the resting phase. With enough hair loss and slow rate of growth, soon the scalp will show through. Starvation depletes the body of important nutrients for the quality of life—let alone hair growth. The long-term effect will lead to reduction in hormone production and can cause other internal issues.

Changing your diet now will affect your hair and your quality of life overall. If your hair has been visibly affected by poor diet, changing your diet will only affect the new growth, not the part of the hair that is already visible. Don't hesitate starting a hair-healthy diet today—although it doesn't mean you will have a beautiful head of hair for another six months to a year, depending on how fast your hair grows.

Hair growth rates vary between about 1/4" and 11/4" per month, contingent upon age, gender, ethnicity, and other genetic and lifestyle factors. This also depends on you caring for your hair properly. On average, a person can expect to have about six inches of new growth every year, so it will take that long to notice the effects of your nutritional changes.

So you are what you eat, and so is your hair.

Vitamins

B Vitamins: Foliate, B6, B12

These important vitamins are involved in creating red blood cells. These blood cells carry oxygen and nutrients to all body cells, including those of the scalp, follicles, and growing hair. Without enough B vitamins, these cells can starve, causing shedding, slow growth, or weak hair that is prone to breaking. If you are not having a problem in these areas, this can help to keep hair strong, healthy, and growing. Can't hurt.

Best Foods for Vitamin B6:

- Acorn
- Apricots
- Avocadoes
- Bananas
- Barley
- Broccoli
- Brussels sprouts
- Butternut
- Carrots
- Chickpeas (garbanzo beans)
- Eggs
- Lean beef
- Lentils
- Oats
- Peanuts and peanut butter
- Peppers
- Pistachio nuts
- Pork tenderloin
- Potatoes (white and sweet)
- Rice (brown, wild)
- Shrimp
- Skinless chicken
- Strawberries
- Tofu
- Tomato paste
- Watermelon
- Whole grain bread
- Wild salmon (fresh, canned)
- Winter squash

Best Foods for Vitamin B12:

- Cheese (fat-free, reduced-fat)
- Cottage cheese (fat-free, 1% low-fat)
- Eggs
- Lean beef
- Milk (fat-free, 1% low-fat)

- Shellfish (clams, oysters, crab)
- Soy milk
- Trout (rainbow, wild)
- Tuna (canned light)
- Veggie burgers
- Wild salmon (fresh, canned)
- Yogurt (fat-free, low-fat)

Best Foods for Folate:

- Artichokes
- Beets
- Berries (boysenberries, blackberries, strawberries)
- Black-eyed peas
- Broccoli
- Broccoli raab
- Brussels sprouts
- Cauliflower
- Chinese cabbage
- Corn
- Green peas
- Lentils
- Mustard greens
- Oats
- Okra
- Oranges and orange juice
- Papaya
- Parsnips
- Seaweed
- Soybeans
- Spinach
- Starchy beans (such as black, navy, pinto, garbanzo, and kidney)
- Sunflower seeds
- Turnip greens
- Wheat germ
- Whole grain bread
- Whole grain pasta

This part of my research was very essential for me personally after I had weight loss surgery in 2002 and later became anemic. Although I had been told to take iron supplements, they just weren't enough.

According to a study completed by Everyday Health (2013) at JoyBaur.com, "Iron helps red blood cells carry oxygen. Iron deficiency can lead to anemia, a condition in which cells don't get enough oxygen to function properly."

This is like suffocating the hair follicles. Anemia leaves the body weak and fatigued and possibly causes hair loss for some women. Most premenopausal women have reported severe hair loss because of low iron reserves. Women who are still in childbearing years are likely to have a deficiency from blood loss during menstruation. Women who have issues with fibroids and tumors may experience a large amount of hair loss because of the large amount of blood loss and the frequency of the loss. Women with heavier flows are more likely to have an iron deficiency than women with less, which will result in more hair loss in those women.

For most people, foods can provide all the iron necessary for good health and strong hair. There are some who will need to take iron supplements to aid in good well being and strong hair. Protein is necessary for all cell growth, especially hair cells, because it's made up of protein. Hair gets its structure from keratin, and without protein for keratin, your strands will weaken and grow slower. This is why shampoos and conditioners with keratin are great!

Here are few that I suggest that you can actually purchase. These are quality products that will give you great results.

- It's A 10
- Chi with Keratin
- Organix Brazilian Keratin

Iron-rich food is also an important part of a hair-healthy diet.

Best Iron-Rich Meats:

- Clams
- Egg yolks
- Lean beef and lamb

- Oysters
- Pork tenderloin
- Shrimp
- Skinless chicken and turkey (especially dark meat)

Best Iron-Rich, High-Protein Vegetables:

- Black-eyed peas
- Lentils
- Soybeans (edamame)
- Starchy beans (such as black, navy, pinto, garbanzo, kidney)
- Tempeh
- Tofu

Best Iron-Rich, Low-Protein Vegetables:

- Asparagus
- Broccoli
- Brussels sprouts
- Kale
- Mustard greens
- Seaweed
- Spinach
- Swiss chard

Beta-Carotene

Beta-carotene in foods is converted to vitamin A in the body. Vitamin A is necessary for all cell growth, including hair cells. A deficiency can lead to dry, dull, lifeless hair and dry skin, which can flake off into dandruff. This can sometimes be confused with a vitamin D deficiency because of the dry and flaky scalp. Note that you can have too much of a good thing when it comes to vitamin A—excessive amounts can cause hair loss. Rather than taking more beta-Carotene, eat more vitamin-A-rich foods rather than taking vitamin A supplements.

Check your vitamin labels like you check your food labels. When buying vitamin A, make sure you only buy 50 percent in the form of retinol. Retinol is listed on supplement labels as palmitate or acetate. The other 50 percent or more should come in the form of beta-Carotene or mixed carotenoids, which are converted to vitamin A only as we need it.

Best Foods for Beta-Carotene:

- Apricots
- Asparagus
- Butternut squash
- Cantaloupe
- Carrots
- Cherries
- Chinese cabbage
- Collard greens
- Grapefruit
- Guava
- Kale
- Lettuce (romaine, green leaf, red leaf, butter head)
- Mangos
- Mustard greens
- Pumpkin
- Red peppers
- Spinach
- Sweet potatoes
- Swiss chard
- Tomatoes
- Turnip greens
- Watercress
- Watermelon

Zinc

The mineral zinc is involved in tissue growth and repair, including hair growth. This helps the oil glands around the follicles to work properly. Low levels of zinc can cause hair loss, slow growth, and dandruff. If these glands aren't working properly, this can cause follicles to be clogged and lead to improper tissue growth, which will result in hair loss.

The amount you get from eating foods rich in zinc is plenty to keep your tresses looking gorgeous. We get enough of this in our regular multivitamin, so there's no need to take excess zinc minerals. The excess inhibits the body's ability to absorb copper.

Best Foods for Zinc:

- Black-eyed peas
- Butter pecans
- Cashews
- Clams
- Crab
- Lean beef
- Lean lamb
- Lentils
- Lima beans
- Lobster
- Mussels
- Ostrich
- Oysters
- Peanuts and peanut butter
- Pine nuts
- Pork tenderloin
- Pumpkin seeds
- Skinless chicken or turkey (especially dark meat)
- Soybeans (edamame)
- Starchy beans (such as black, navy, pinto, garbanzo, kidney)
- Sunflower seeds
- Wheat germ
- Yogurt (fat-free, low-fat)

Exercise

Most conditions that affect your health show up through your hair. In most cases, if your medical condition will allow you to exercise and boost your overall health, then it will reflect that in your hair. (Anything that affects your bloodstream is going to affect your hair.)

What better way to increase blood flow to the entire body faster than by exercising? It can be just a simple walk around the block to bring more blood flow to the body rather than being sedentary. Think about it: a person who's donating blood may be given a ball to squeeze as a way of increasing flow. This quickly increases blood flow to the veins. If you have not worked out lately, start out with walking. Just get moving!

Working out improves blood circulation, according to the American Heart Association. Get more physical activity into your life through exercises; yoga is listed as one of the best ways to improve blood circulation to your scalp, according to Holistic Online. Increased scalp circulation will stimulate hair follicles, causing hair growth.

Metabolism

This section is important here because it goes right along with diet and exercise. Many of us don't do these two things together properly, which sends our metabolism into shock. We are not aware that this affects our hair.

Metabolism is best described as the process in which the body burns energy. Everything we do requires the use of energy, including sleeping. Dieting can be very detrimental to the metabolism if not done properly. Most people end up taking in too few calories to sustain the body. This is when hair loss occurs.

How much and how often you eat is important when you want to boost your metabolism. When we don't take in enough food, our body goes into starvation mode. The best thing to do is to eat several small meals four to five times a day, which keeps your metabolism boosted throughout the day.

Water is another important element; it also helps you to feel full. Dehydration slows down the metabolism because you feel tired and lifeless. Drink at least sixty-four ounces of water a day for recommended daily intake; but to maximize, drink half your body weight in ounces.

Supplements

One of the most important vitamins for hair health is *biotin*. This is actually a form of vitamin B that is widely used to help prevent hair loss and stimulate hair growth. It is often recommended for chemotherapy patients to help increase the rate of growth.

This vitamin is also useful for thinning hair and is thought to help with loss of hair pigmentation, although no conclusive evidence has been found. Biotin helps our bodies to break down fats, protein, and carbohydrates. Because of the breakdown, some people have noticed weight loss when taking it. Biotin is also found in some foods naturally, which most people are unaware of. It can be found in Swiss chard, liver, halibut, and goat milk, to name a few.

Several other B vitamins help with hair loss. Panthenol, or vitamin B5, is often used externally in shampoos and other hair products to help increase thickness. It has the ability to penetrate the cuticle and increase the diameter as a topical supplement. But if your hair is naturally thin, then there is nothing that is actually going to make it thicker—only things that make it appear fuller.

A deficiency of vitamin B12 can lead to anemia, which stunts hair growth. This almost has the same effects as low iron when it comes to anemia. Supplements of this vitamin often fall short, as they don't absorb very well. Vitamin B12 shots are given for energy support in those who are deficient. However, you can also increase your levels of this vitamin by eating foods like grass-fed beef, egg yolks, and free-range poultry.

Antioxidant vitamins are also an important source of nutrition for healthy hair. Vitamins C, E, and A are important for the health of the skin and hair. That is why you see excess growth with vitamins that have all these included together. They help promote healthy connective tissues and cellular growth. A diet rich in these vitamins provides support for vibrant, abundant hair growth. Vitamin E also increases scalp circulation, which in turn promotes hair growth, which is very important for recovering chemotherapy patients.

Hydration

Anyone who has ever sat in my chair can tell you that this is my favorite topic of all time. I can notice right away if a client is not hydrated because it shows right through her hair. Look at it this way: You are a plant that needs to be watered, and without it, the leaves turn yellow and brown and they fall off the tree. That's why when they drug test, they take a strand of hair, because those toxins tend to stay in your hair. If you are not properly hydrating your body with the recommended six to eight glasses a day, then you are barely flushing your vital organs, so there's no chance of any making it to your hair. (It is impossible to have healthy hair and not drink water.)

An average adult body is made up of at least forty-two liters of water with a loss of about 2.7. He can suffer from dehydration. Some of the symptoms range from fatigue, nervousness, dizziness, irritability, weakness, and headaches and can reach a state of pathology. In a book by Dr. F. Batmanghelidj, it states that our body cries out for water. The symptoms listed are warning signs before you ultimately faint.

If your hair is shedding due to dehydration, no amount of conditioners or protein will do the trick. There are many benefits to drinking water and staying properly hydrated. Everything starts from the inside out. Even having healthier looking hair!

Chapter 4: Things That Could Affect Your Hair Growth

Now that I have given what I believe to be the proper tools to grow out your hair, I think it is just as important that I share some things that could *affect* your hair growth. Some of these things you may or may not have control over, but I shared these things with my clients and it has helped them on their healthy hair journey.

Environmental Influences

A 2008 "Environmental Influences on Gene Expressions" study on Nature Education by Ingrid Lobo, PhD shows that certain drugs and chemicals in the environments cause hair loss.

According to a website called Blackmold, if you live in a house with a mold problem, you could start to lose your hair. The allergic reactions humans suffer from mold can lead to hair loss. The roots of your hair are nourished by tiny blood vessels called *capillaries*. If the circulation to these blood vessels is disrupted, the hair can fall out or break. The same would happen if you had a disruption in blood flow in other areas of your body.

When you breathe in mold spores, they trigger allergic reactions in your body. During these allergic reactions, your immune system creates a chemical called *histamine*. The histamine causes inflammation, which disrupts the blood flow in the capillaries. This leads to the hairs not getting enough blood and eventually falling out. (Remember here again: anything that affects your bloodstream will affect your hair.)

There are other things mold can affect health-wise. If you suspect you have been exposed to mold, please seek medical attention immediately. This type of hair loss can be restored.

Once the person is no longer exposed to mold and the follicles are not dead, there's a chance for hair restoration. Treatments should not be delayed, because once the follicle dies, hair cannot be restored. The person has to be treated for fungal infection because this type of infection is contagious.

Street Drugs

There are some street drugs that have been linked to hair loss, such as methamphetamine and cocaine use. It has been stated that meth and cocaine use takes a toll on appearance; continued use can lead to rotting teeth due to poor hygiene and bacterial buildup.

Due to the high acidity in the drugs, they can lead to tooth decay. Additionally, due to the toxic chemicals that are found in meth, hair loss is also something that is common among users both long term and short term. This type of hair loss will take time and some cleansing, healthy living, and a wholesome lifestyle, but it can regrow once a person returns to a healthy state.

Testosterone (DHT)

Having high testosterone for men is considered a good thing but not so much for women. For men, it gives them a high sex drive. This could also be true for women, but there is a certain level that will make your hair shed.

Too much exercise is actually bad for your hair. Excessive exercise causes a state of chronic stress in your body, according to author and nutritionist Ann Louise Gittleman. Chronic stress is a leading cause of telogen effluvium (TE), a condition that causes premature resting and shedding in hair follicles, according to the American Hair Loss Association. Over exercising can produce more dihydrotestosterone (DHT), which causes male-pattern baldness. But on the other hand, mild exercise, like regular jogging or cardio, can help reduce DHT. This is a form of hair loss that depends on the level of testosterone and whether it will regrow to its once-healthy state.

Another thing to keep in mind about exercise is that it causes you to sweat. Salty, heavy sweat buildup on your head can cause faster shedding or further damage to your hair. The Harvard School of Public Health advises that you combat this damage by using mild, pH-balanced shampoo and moisturizing protein conditioner at least once a week

For already-thinning hair, try thickening shampoo and volumizing conditioner to help combat hair loss and stimulate hair regrowth. Avoid using hot hair tools as well, such as blow dryers and curling irons after workouts. Heat should never be reapplied to your hair once you have sweat buildup; it should be freshly shampooed before applying heat. This is damaging to your hair. If you must blow dry, use the dryer on its cool setting.

Tinea Capitis (Ringworm)

Tinea capitis is the scientific name for ringworm on the scalp. This is most common in children, especially ages three to seven. The fungi produces spores that shed into the infected child's clothing, brushes, and even into the air around the child. These spores can survive for months on objects.

Children and barbers who don't properly clean tools are more likely to pass ringworms on than anyone else. It is even possible to pass ringworms on to our animals if we are not careful.

The most common symptom is hair loss. There is also a rash, which can look different depending on whether the fungus gets inside the hair shaft or stays on the outside of the hair shaft. If not treated right away, the infected area will spread and hair loss will take a very long time to grow back. Some have noticed at least a year.

It is important to note that it cannot be treated with antifungal topical creams. It has to be treated with oral antifungal medications, sometimes for several months.

Bacterial Folliculitis

Folliculitis is an infection in the hair follicles. The infection can occur due to exposure to fungi, a virus, or bacteria entering the skin. This type of follicle infection can be caused by too-tight weaves, braids, or pulling from the scalp. This also can happen from leaving the weave in too long and receiving a fungus from bacteria.

A bacterial folliculitis infection can involve the superficial layers of skin of the follicle, or may cause symptoms deep in the skin layers and affect the whole hair follicle, according to the Mayo Clinic. Folliculitis caused by bacteria may require a trip to the doctor for proper treatment if the condition does not resolve quickly.

Red bumps appear at the hair follicle, and the skin surrounding the area is inflamed and reddened. This can happen from double-dipping wax from salons or dirty tools scraping the skin. It is very important to sanitize implements.

Possible complications of bacterial folliculitis include an increased spread of the infection to surrounding hair follicles and permanent hair loss due to the damage sustained by the follicle.

Chapter 5: Understanding Everyone's Role

Stylist's Role

As a stylist, not only have I realized I'm responsible for making sure that I'm using good-quality products on my clients, but I am also responsible for researching and understanding the products I'm using.

The client comes into the salon fully entrusting the stylist with her hair-care needs (most of them, anyway). Some can do their own hair; they just need our hands. So as a professional, it is my responsibility to care for my client's hair on my watch. Now if the client is cheating me—going to more than one hairstylist—that is a hard case. I handle with caution.

In my research in the last ten years, I have noticed a fair amount of women who have been dissatisfied with their last stylist. The client often states either the stylist was responsible for her hair loss or did not know how to stop her hair from coming out. I believe the client feels this way due to a lack of knowledge on both parts. There could have been several reasons why she was losing her hair, but because it went unaddressed, it was believed to be the stylist's fault.

I once met a client who told me her last stylist was responsible for her hair loss. She came into the salon, and I gave her a consultation. I asked all the questions: How much water are you drinking? Are you on medication? What kind of shampoo and conditioner do you use?

She stated, "Oh, I don't drink water."

Well, there's your problem. I told her, "You can go back to your stylist. It's not her fault. If you come to me and continue not drinking water, you're going to have the same issue."

By the time the client makes it to my chair, she is hurt and looking for answers and not very trusting. I have always tried to make it a point to never bad-mouth another hair-care professional, because it would only make me look unprofessional and the client will feel uneasy. My goal is to get them to relax, talk to me, tell me about their hair (not the stylist), give me some background information that's going to help me track down the issue, and come up with a solution. Being knowledgeable in my craft has helped my business.

For instance, when a lawyer passes the bar, he does not stop studying the law because he does not know all the old laws. Also, the laws are continuing to change and there are new ones being created every day. But I have found that in the beauty industry, there are more classes to update you on styling, cutting, and color than knowledge of healthiness in the field. We as hair-care professionals must seek it out for ourselves.

As stylists, we sometimes do things that we aren't necessarily good at, and this hurts us in the long run instead of focusing more on what we are good at doing. I wanted to do healthy hair, so I began the research to expand my knowledge into what would make me better in the market at what I was already inspired to do. So instead of charging extra for deep conditioners, hot oil treatments, and protein packs like everyone, I gave them away for free. Did it hurt sometimes? Of course it did, but I stayed busy most of the time and it balanced out. I thought it was redundant to say I specialized in healthy hair and then charge someone to make it healthy. This made me stand out from my competition. The funny thing is: some of them never even saw me as competition. I loved it this way!

As a professional, I feel I have a duty to my clients to show up on time, not keep them waiting for hours, not forget their appointments, and to keep a professional environment as much as possible.

Today's stylists have left a bad taste in the mouth of so many clients because they fail to give them good customer service. Some think because we are self-employed we don't have to answer to anyone. Well, we do! We answer to the clients who don't return because they don't appreciate the way they have been treated. I would hope that stylists would get better with showing their customers they appreciate them. People who pay for a service want to know they are appreciated. No one wants to continue to patronize with someone who is rude and unappreciative. I make it a conscious effort to remember that they are my business and I am here to serve them.

Client's Role

The client's role is just as important as the stylist's because this is teamwork. If you are a person without a stylist, then your role is solo. You can still follow the same guidelines; you're just going at it alone. As a client, depending on how often you go into the salon—whether it is once a week, every two weeks, or every six to eight weeks for your relaxer and trim, or every blue moon—you are with you more than the stylist is with you.

So that means: the majority of the responsibility of the maintenance falls on you. This is a very important part of the process. The way you care for your hair in between your services; drinking your water; if you are on a vitamin regimen; wrapping your hair at night; not applying too much heat. Follow the directions of your stylist and ask questions when you need to.

If you have a stylist or if you are in search of one, talk to them about medications, medical issues, and upcoming surgeries.

If you are in need of a stylist, you should be interviewing the stylist to know if they are a fit for you or not. Taking in to consideration hours of operation, specialties, religious preferences, driving distance, even age, and prices. This way, you're not chair-hopping every month with your hair. Sometimes these things are often overlooked; and sometimes they just don't matter when you have found a great stylist by referral.

Also, as a client, it is your duty to cancel an appointment and avoid being a no-show. Stylists do not get any vacation time or leave. So we need to be able to reschedule other clients, but we can only do this with advance notice.

Purpose of Using Quality Products

Stylist

As a stylist, when I'm purchasing products for my clients, it makes me feel good as a stylist to know that I'm using the best. I've learned to gather more information about those products beforehand, taking notice of some of the ingredients in the product and what's going to give me the best results. Knowing which shampoo to use helps also. For example, a clarifying (cleansing) versus a moisturizing for a client who works out a lot and has sweat buildup. If one of the first four ingredients is alcohol, then it is too much for African-American hair.

If the client's hair is already building acid from working out—which dries out the hair—you definitely don't want to add more alcohol to the hair. I normally use a cleansing shampoo to remove the buildup, followed by a moisturizing shampoo.

On the product label, whatever ingredients are first, the product contains more of; whatever ingredients are last, the product contains less of.

I never wanted the line of products that I used in the salon to be something that my clients could go into the beauty supply and purchase. One reason is that it makes them feel as if they can do what you do with the product, even though they cannot. The other is: if they are going to a salon professional, they should be getting professional products. I want the client to feel as though they cannot get the same look at home that they could achieve at the salon; one reason is because of the products. Investing in quality products is worth it. Not expensive products, but quality products.

Here's a list of quality products that aren't too expensive. These products are also versatile; they can be used on any race.

- Organix
- KeraCare
- Chi
- Biosilk

Client

As a client purchasing products, always talk to your stylist if you have one. Even if you don't, you can always walk into a salon and buy quality products from a salon. You don't have to purchase products just from the shelves anymore. But it all depends on what you are looking for too; some things you may have to go to the beauty supply store to find.

The main products you should be purchasing from the salon are your shampoos, conditioners, oils, and hairsprays. The other styling agents are really at your discretion, and it depends on what type of hair you have and what you are trying to achieve. If you want great results, you need to purchase quality products. It starts at the beginning with a great shampoo and conditioner.

If you have natural (chemical-free) hair, you should be using non-sulfate with keratin shampoo and conditioners to ensure moisture and strength. If you are relaxed, I suggest moisturizing shampoo and conditioner to retain that hair keeps its moisture, luster, and shine.

Again, I emphasize that the products do not have to be expensive to be of good quality. But you cannot buy a quality hair product from the dollar store. If achieving healthy hair is your goal, you are going to have to spend a few extra dollars.

Chapter 6: Unmasking a Woman's Hidden Beauty

Personal Changes and Influences

There are so many reasons that women step into a beauty salon; whether it's to keep their hair up because it makes them feel good, or for work, their mate, for show, the Joneses, a date, special occasion, or whatever the reason may be. The reason they are getting it done at that point and time is special to them; sometimes they mark a personal change in their life. Again, professionals have the opportunity to wave their wand and make a transformation or a tragedy in the lives of everyday women.

Maybe everyday plain Jane, who gets the same old hairstyle, is thinking of getting something a little different. The stylist may not be paying attention or decided to do her own thing. Because sometimes stylists can totally just go way out of the box, depending on how creative they may be feeling that day, it's possible Jane will not be happy with her new style. She now has something that she hates and makes her feel uncomfortable. It's a beautiful style, but just not for Jane. (That's what we call a *tragedy*.)

On the other hand, a stylist has the ability to wave the wand and do what Jane asks for. You know her as a client; you know she just wants something slightly different, but not too much flash. She's even open to suggestions, because she trusts your input. She loves the idea, and her new style is great. She is happy and she's feeling like a new women. (And that's a *transformation*.)

I have the ability to wave the magic wand and make a transformation or a tragedy. But there's a rewarding feeling from being a part of the transformation and unmasking the hidden beauty inside of so many women, watching their faces change with the feeling they get from a great style that they love.

How a Salon Visit Can Affect Self-Esteem

This runs hand-in-hand with the previous section. What the client ends up with upon leaving your salon can ultimately affect their self-esteem. I know for some of you, you may be thinking, *How is this even possible?* Believe me—it is!

As the client, they have their mind fixed on one thing they want, but sometimes as stylists, we have grown accustom to doing it our way (but without telling the client). The client is the one who has to wear it and the ultimate decision is theirs on the style they receive.

In our industry, we have so much freedom of expression because we are creating art. We must be careful that the canvas that's being created on is open to the idea. If not, then we want to ensure there is humility on our part to allow clients to feel just as free to express their unhappiness.

I want to have a friendly business relationship with open dialogue with my clients where she knows her opinion is respected and business is appreciated. But it took years of practice and many losses of good clients to get to this point. When they leave the salon, they don't feel belittled and scorned in front of other clients. I had to learn to be approachable and open to constructive criticism. They will want to be repeat clients and refer others.

Bad Haircut Can Be Disastrous

Whether the haircut was thought out or on impulse by the client, if it's not what's expected, it could end in disaster. Make sure before giving a haircut that you have talked to the client and they have shown you a picture of what they want the haircut to look like. This cuts down on unexpected results from the client.

Being a professional and just totally giving a client a cut that she did not ask for or did not expect could be the end of that relationship. Most times, a person has to mentally prepare for a haircut before getting one, or it at least has to be their decision.

I have said so many times and I will say it one last time: I have the ability to wave a magic wand and make a transformation or a tragedy. But one thing we cannot do is wave our wand and put hair back on—only weave it.

So when it comes to cutting, we must be very careful on how we handle this part of our business. I particularly do not cut any client without a consultation and a picture. If it's a client who has shared with me that she wants her hair to grow out, I will ask her to think about it and let me know on the next visit. If she still wants it done, then I will cut it for her. If it's a client going from really long to really short, I ask her to go halfway and think about it before going completely short to see how she feels with the shorter hair. Then if she wants more cut, I will give her the next cut for free.

As Beautiful as She Feels

As a stylist, it is considered a blessing and an honor when I get a client and a head of hair. I receive them at first knowing that they could have stopped at hundreds of salons before they came to me. I recognize that the clients are the heart and soul of the business and that they trust me with one of their most prized possessions: their hair.

We have made the statement for years that our hair is our glory. So ask yourself: why would you allow just anyone in it? You cannot! It has to be someone you trust. A woman is only as beautiful as she feels. This starts from the inside out. No matter how much a man tells a woman she is beautiful, if she does not feel that way, she will not believe him. If a woman's self-esteem is low, then she will not feel beautiful even if she is. A stylist has a way to help a woman bring out this inner beauty just from styling her hair, from their conversations they have in the salon, and even from the atmosphere.

In my salon atmosphere, I have created a positive environment. A sisterhood, a bond, where women can network and make connections. There is so much negativity already going on outside the salon that I want to make their salon experience a positive one.

I have been given a gift to recognize that from the atmosphere in the salon to the conversations I hold with my clients to the music I play, I'm speaking into the lives of every woman who enters my door, whether I know it or not. This place can be used as a negative or a positive. Every chance I get, I use it as a positive influence in the lives of others.

I have had so many woman come back to me and tell me how blessed they were in my salon because of the atmosphere—not because it was the most up-to-date but because of the peace and the conversation. They said it was one of the first salons they went to where there was no gossiping and they felt that I truly cared for the health of their hair. Women have poured out their hearts and souls to me, given their lives to Christ, prayed with me, and I've even taken a client into my home who was being abused.

What I aspire for every woman to know that enters into Something Special Styling Salon in Irving, Texas, is that they are special to me, to God, and they should be to themselves. I want to help them see the beauty that is lying dormant on the inside of them that's been hidden way too long. For some women, this is not an issue and we just form a sisterhood, but for some, it's way overdue.

I feel as though I have fulfilled my obligation spiritually and ethically to my clients, and now I have shared with others.

References

"Environmental Influences on Gene Expressions" (2008). Nature Education by: Ingrid Lobo, PhD.

"When Hair Loss Is Not Genetic" (2011). Krisha McCoy; medically reviewed by Lindsey Marcellin, MD, MPH.

"The Biology of Hair Follicles" (1999). Paus, Ralif; Cotsarelis, George, the *New England Journal of Medicine*.

"Controls of Hair Follicle Cycling" (2001). K. S. Stenn; Paus, Ralif, *Physiological Reviews.*

"Anagen Phase, Telogen Phase, and Catagen Phase" (2007). Brannon, Maryland, Heather, *The New York Times.*

WebMD, 2005–2013

Dr. Daniel K. Hall-Flavin, MD

Revivogen.com

The University of Maryland Medical Center

Everyday Health (2013) at JoyBaur.com

American Heart Association

American Hair Loss Association

The Harvard School of Public Health

Importance of Water